I0449237

The Ultimate Guide on Safe Use of Essential Oils

ISBN 978-1-300-81262-3
Christoffer Kilbourne

TABLE OF CONTENT

CHAPTER 1

INTRODUCTION

What Do Essential Oils Mean?

Essential oils are products from plants that are very concentrated and have the natural scent and health benefits of the plant they come from. The most common ways to get these oils are through cold pressing or steam distillation. Essential oils are made from the essence of different parts of plants, like flowers, leaves, stems, bark, and roots. The chemicals that make up each essential oil are different, which is what gives them their unique smell and may help with health problems. For example, chemicals like linalool and linalyl acetate in lavender oil are known to calm people down. Peppermint oil, on the other hand, is known for its energizing smell and cooling effect because it is high in menthol.

Use in the past and popularity

Essential oils have been used for thousands of years. People in old times knew they could be used for both healing and scenting. Essential oils were very important in ancient Egypt for both mummification and daily beauty and health routines. Egyptian writings talk about how oils like myrrh, frankincense, and cedarwood were used. These oils were highly valued for their ability to keep things fresh and smell good.

In ancient Greece, experts like Hippocrates and Theophrastus wrote a lot about how medicinal plants could help with health problems. The Greeks took what the Egyptians knew and built on it. They used oils for spiritual, medical, and beauty uses. In the same way, essential oils were used in baths, massages, and medical treatments every day in ancient Rome. The Romans, who were known for being very wealthy, used these oils as part of their complicated beauty and hygiene practices.

People in Asia were also affected by essential oils. Traditional Chinese medicine and Indian Ayurvedic medicine used these natural products to treat illnesses. In India, for example, oils like sandalwood and neem have been used for hundreds of years to heal a wide range of illnesses and make religious ceremonies more powerful.

Essential oils were valued in the Middle Ages because they killed germs, especially during times of plague and other widespread diseases. Essential oils kept being used in new ways. In the early 1900s, French chemist René-Maurice Gattefossé came up with the name aromatherapy after finding that lavender oil could help heal burns.

In modern times, essential oils have become very famous. People all over the world use these natural remedies for a wide range of concerns. Essential oils are used by many people who are looking for natural and holistic answers for everything from cleaning and aromatherapy to skin care and wellness. Why safe practices are important

Essential oils have many benefits, but it is very important to use them correctly to avoid any bad effects. Because these oils are concentrated, they are strong and can hurt you if you don't use them right. People who use essential oils can get the benefits without putting their health and well-being at risk by following safe practices.

Proper Diluting: One of the most important safety steps is to make sure that essential oils are diluted correctly before putting them on your skin. If you don't reduce oils, they can irritate, sensitize, or even burn your skin. By mixing the essential oil with a carrier oil like coconut oil, jojoba oil, or almond oil, you can make it safer and lower the chance of side effects. There are different dilution amounts needed for different oils and uses, so it is important to follow the instructions that are specific to the oil and use.

Patch Testing: It is best to do a patch test before using a new essential oil. To do this, a small amount of diluted oil should be put on a hidden part of the skin, like the inside of the forearm, and the person should watch for 24 to 48 hours for any signs of irritation or an allergic response. Patch testing helps find out which parts of the body are sensitive and makes sure the oil is safe to use on bigger areas.

Storage: Another important part of safe use is storing essential oils the right way. Keep essential oils in dark glass bottles to keep them safe from light, which can break down their quality over time. Don't put them near heat sources and make sure kids and pets can't get to them. Keep them somewhere cool and dry. Keeping oils in the right way helps them keep working well.

Methods of Application: There are different safety issues that need to be thought about for each method of application. For example, if you want to use essential oils in an aromatherapy device, make sure there is enough air flow and only use the right amount of oils so that they don't overpower your senses. Things like the eyes and mucous tissues should be kept away from when oils are applied to the skin. Additionally, some essential oils are not safe to take by mouth and should never be done so without the supervision of a trained medical professional.

Special Populations: Pregnant women, babies, and pets are all vulnerable groups that should be especially careful when using essential oils. Some oils may not be good for these groups, so they should use them less or not at all. For these people, talking to a doctor or an expert aromatherapist can help them figure out how to use it safely.

CHAPTER 2

Understanding Essential Oils

Composition of Chemicals

Essential oils are made up of a lot of different volatile compounds that give them their smell and healing qualities. Terpenes, esters, alcohols, aldehydes, ketones, phenols, and oxides make up most of these substances. There is a unique mix of these chemicals in each essential oil, which gives each one its own flavor and health benefits.

These are the most common chemicals that can be found in essential oils. Based on how many isoprene units they have, they can be put into three groups: monoterpenes, sesquiterpenes, and diterpenes. Some of the health benefits of terpenes are that they reduce inflammation, kill germs, and fight viruses. One monoterpene found in citrus oils is limonene, which is known for its ability to make people feel better and kill germs.

Esters: An alcohol and an acid combine to make an ester. Most of the time, they smell nice and sweet, and they are known to calm and reduce inflammation. Linalyl acetate is a common ester that is found in lavender oil and is known to help people sleep.

These chemicals are called alcohols because they have a hydroxyl group (-OH) linked to a carbon atom. They're usually not too strong, and they can kill germs, viruses, and fungi. One example is menthol, which can be found in peppermint oil and can cool you down and ease pain.

A carbonyl group (C=O) is linked to a hydrogen atom in an aldehyde. A lot of the time, they smell strong and can be bad for your face. They do, however, have important antimicrobial and anti-inflammatory qualities. An aldehyde is something like citral, which is found in lemongrass oil.

There is also a carbonyl group in ketones, but it is connected to two carbon atoms. They are known for their ability to dissolve mucus and repair damaged tissue. One example is the gastric aid carvone, which can be found in spearmint oil.

It is made up of phenols, which have a hydroxyl group attached straight to an aromatic hydrocarbon group. They kill germs very well, but they can be irritating to the skin and mucous tissues. The chemical thymol, which is found in thyme oil, is a well-known antiseptic.

Oxides: Oxides are made up of two or more elements that are bound together. A lot of the time, they help with breathing problems because they make you cough. Eucalyptus oil contains 1,8-cineole, a common acid that is known to help clear up stuffy noses.

Knowing the chemicals that make up essential oils can help you figure out what benefits they might have and how to use them safely. The therapeutic qualities and right uses of each oil depend on its own unique mix of compounds.
Types of Essential Oils You May Know

Lavender (Lavandula angustifolia): Lavender oil is often used to help people relax and sleep, relieve stress, and heal skin irritations because it is known to be peaceful and calming. Linalool and linalyl acetate are the main chemicals that make it up.

Melaleuca alternifolia, or tea tree, oil is known for being very good at killing germs and fungi. It is often used in skin care products to treat acne, fungus infections, and small cuts and scrapes. Terpinen-4-ol and alpha-terpineol are its main active ingredients.

Peppermint (Mentha piperita): Peppermint oil is often used to treat headaches, improve focus, and ease stomach problems because it wakes you up and cools you down. Menthol and menthone are the main ingredients in it.

Eucalyptus (Eucalyptus globulus): Eucalyptus oil is known to help the lungs and is used to clear up stuffy noses, ease coughs, and clear up congestion. 1,8-cineole, also known as eucalyptol, is its main ingredient.

Lemon (Citrus limon): Lemon oil is used to improve mood, support immune system function, and clean surfaces because it makes people feel good and cleans. Limonene is the main ingredient in it.

Frankincense (Boswellia carteri): Frankincense oil is used in meditation, on the skin, and to boost the immune system. It is thought to help you feel grounded and refreshed. Alpha-pinene and other sesquiterpenes are its main parts.

Chamomile (Matricaria chamomilla): Chamomile oil is used to help people relax, treat skin problems, and lower inflammation because it is known to calm and reduce inflammation. Chamazulene and bisabolol are two of its main ingredients.

Rosemary (Rosmarinus officinalis): Rosemary oil is used to improve focus, help hair grow, and ease muscle pain. It is valued for its ability to stimulate and improve memory. 1,8-cineole, camphor, and alpha-pinene are some of its main parts.

Knowing about these common types of essential oils and what they are mostly made of helps people choose the right oils for their wants and uses.
Different ways to extract

The way that essential oils are extracted can have a big effect on their quality, effectiveness, and healing qualities. Steam distillation, cold pressing, solvent extraction, and CO2 extraction are some of the most popular ways to get something out of plants.

Steam distillation is the most common way to get essential oils out of plants. The essential oil is turned into gas when steam is passed through the plant matter.

The oil and steam fumes are then cooled and collected, which separates the oil from the water. Herb, leaf, and flower oils, like those from lavender, peppermint, and eucalyptus, are often made by steam distillation.

Cold pressing: This method is mostly used to get oils out of citrus fruits like orange, lemon, and bergamot. In this method, the essential oil is released by pressing the fruit peel with a machine. After this, the oil is removed from the juice and other parts. The delicate aromatic chemicals are kept safe during cold pressing, which makes high-quality oils that smell good.

Solvent Extraction: Flowers and plants that are too fragile to handle the high temperatures of steam distillation are used for solvent extraction. Solvents like hexane or ethanol are used in this method to separate the essential oil from the plant matter. The liquid is then lost, leaving only the oil that has been concentrated. Rose and jasmine oils are made this way. But very small amounts of the solvent may still be in the finished product, which some people may not like.

CO2 Extraction: This is a new way to get essential oils out of plants by using supercritical CO_2, which is carbon dioxide at a very high pressure and very low temperature. It dissolves the essential oil from the plant matter because CO2 is a solvent. The pressure is then lowered, and the CO2 turns back into a gas. The pure essential oil is left behind. Some oils, like frankincense and chamomile, are made with this method, which makes them very good and full of different aromatic chemicals.

You choose which extraction method to use based on the type of plant material you have and the quality of essential oil you want to make. Understanding these steps helps people understand how hard and carefully it is to make good essential oils.

CHAPTER 3

General Safety Guidelines

Why proper dilution is important

It is very important to dilute essential oils correctly so that they don't cause bad responses like skin irritation, sensitization, or toxicity. When you put essential oils on your face or use them in large amounts, they can have bad effects because they are highly concentrated plant extracts. When you dilute an essential oil, you mix it with a carrier oil to make it less strong and safe to use.

Skin Sensitivity: If you put essential oils on your skin without diluting them, they can irritate it or cause allergic responses. This is especially important for older people, children, and people with sensitive skin. By spreading the essential oil over a bigger area and making it less strong, proper dilution helps lower these risks.

Absorption Through the Skin: Essential oils get into the bloodstream when they are absorbed through the skin. Using oils that aren't diluted raises the risk of systemic toxicity. This is especially true for oils that contain compounds like phenols or ketones, which can be dangerous in large amounts. Dilution makes sure that only a small amount of oil gets into the bloodstream, which is safe.

Instructions for Use: The suggested dilution amounts change based on the essential oil being used and the purpose for which it is being used. A 2-3% dilution (2–3 drops of essential oil per teaspoon of carrier oil) is usually safe for people to use on their skin. For use on the face or on skin that is sensitive, a smaller concentration of 0.5 to 1% is suggested. Higher concentrations (up to 10%) can be used for specific uses, like treating muscle pain, but they should be used with care.

Age Factors: Because they are more sensitive, children, pregnant women, and the old need lower dilution ratios. Diluting it with 0.5 to 1% is usually best for kids, but pregnant women should talk to their doctor or nurse for the right advice. To keep their skin from getting irritated, older people may also benefit from lower reduction ratios.

How to Pick the Best Carrier Oil

Carrier oils are vegetable oils that are used to thin out essential oils before they are put on the skin. They help the essential oil get into the skin better, spread it out, and lower the risk of discomfort. Picking the right carrier oil relies on your skin type, the therapeutic effects you want, and your own personal taste.

Most common carrier oils are:

Coconut Oil: Coconut oil is good for all skin kinds and has a mild, pleasant smell. It is known for moisturizing. When it hits your skin, it melts. It is solid at room temperature.

Jojoba Oil: Because it is similar to the skin's natural sebum, jojoba oil is great for people with oily or acne-prone skin. It doesn't cause acne and helps keep oil production in check.

Sweet Almond Oil: Sweet almond oil is good for dry or sensitive skin because it is full of vitamins A and E. This stuff is light and soaks in fast.

Grapeseed Oil: Grapeseed oil is great for oily or mixed skin because it is light and easy to absorb. It doesn't smell like anything and is full of vitamins.

Olive Oil: Olive oil is good for dry and old skin because it is rich and nourishing. It does, however, smell stronger and be thicker, which some people may not like. Skin Type and Preferences: To get the most out of the essential oil blend, it's important to choose a carrier oil that is good for your skin type. For instance, people with dry skin might like how olive or sweet almond oil moisturizes deeply, while people with oily skin might like how grapeseed or jojoba oil feels lighter on the skin. When picking a carrier oil, you should also think about what you like in terms of smell and feel.

healing Properties: Some carrier oils have healing properties of their own that can work with essential oils to make them more effective. For example, calendula oil is good for soothing skin that is itchy because it reduces inflammation and speeds up the mending process.

Putting on a Patch Test

A patch test is an important way to make sure that an essential oil blend is safe to use and won't irritate or cause an allergic response. This easy test can help people figure out which essential oils make them sensitive.

Here's how to do a patch test:

Prepare the Dilution: Mix the essential oil with a carrier oil in the right amount (for people, 2-3% is a good range).

Apply a Small Amount: Put a little of the diluted oil on a skin spot that won't be seen, like the inside of your wrist or behind your ear.

Watch and Wait: After 24 to 48 hours, keep an eye on the area for any signs of redness, itching, swelling, or other discomfort.

Findings: The essential oil blend is probably safe to use on a larger area of skin if no bad effects happen. If there is any irritation or an allergic response, the oil should be washed off right away, and the blend shouldn't be used.

Important Notes: It is very important to do a patch test before using a new essential oil or a new blend for the first time. Also, it's a good idea to do a patch test before putting oils on sensitive skin or people who already know they have sensitive skin.

Safe Ways to Store and Handle

The right way to store and handle essential oils is very important for keeping them safe, effective, and potent.

If you don't store something properly, it can oxidize, break down, and lose some of its therapeutic effects.

Conditions for storage:

Dark Glass Bottles: Aromatherapy oils should be kept in amber or cobalt blue dark glass bottles to keep them safe from light, which can make them less effective.

Put essential oils somewhere cool and dry, out of the sun, away from heat sources, and out of the way of moist air. Usually, a temperature range of 5 to 20°C (41 to 68°F) is best.

Airtight Seals: Make sure the bottles are tightly sealed so that the essential oils don't oxidize or evaporate. The therapeutic qualities of the oils can be lost if they are exposed to air.

Shelf Life: The shelf life of essential oils depends on what they are made of. Some oils, like citrus oils, go bad faster and only last about one to two years. Other oils, like patchouli and sandalwood, can last for many years. Managing the shelf life well can be done by keeping track of when the oils were bought and using the oldest ones first.
Care When Handling:

To keep from getting contaminated, don't touch the dropper or bottle hole with your fingers or anything else when you're using essential oils.

Childproof storage: Keep essential oils out of reach of kids and pets so they don't accidentally touch or eat them. Using caps that are safe for kids can add an extra layer of safety.

Labeling: Write the names and purchase dates of all essential oil bottles clearly on the labels to keep things clear and make sure they are used correctly.

Properly get rid of essential oils that have gone bad or are past their expiration date. Do not pour them down the drain because they can hurt plants and animals in water. Instead, call the local garbage disposal authority to get advice on how to safely get rid of the trash.

CHAPTER 4

Application Methods

Topical Application
Topical application of essential oils
means putting diluted essential oils on
the skin. This lets the body absorb and
use the good chemicals in the oils.
People like this method because it works
well on specific areas, like relieving
muscle pain, improving skin health, or
giving localized comfort. To make sure
the product works well and safely, you
should know the right reduction ratios,
places to stay away from, and how often
you should use it.
Rates of Dilution for Different Age
Groups

1. Adults:

For general use, a dilution ratio of 2% to
3% is good for most people. To do this,
mix 10 to 15 drops of essential oil with
30 milliliters of neutral oil. This dilution
can be used for massage, general skin
care, and other uses that touch the skin.

Face: The skin on your face is more
sensitive than skin on other parts of your
body. It is suggested to dilute it less,
between 0.5 and 1%, which equals 3 to

6 drops of essential oil per ounce of neutral oil. This helps keep the skin from becoming irritated or sensitive.

For localized treatments, like muscle pain or bug bites, a stronger concentration of up to 10% can be used. For every ounce of neutral oil, this is the same as 50 drops of essential oil. But this should only be used in small places and not very often.

2. Kids:

Babies (0–6 months): Babies younger than six months should not usually be exposed to essential oils. As little as 0.1% to 0.2%, or about 1-2 drops per ounce of neutral oil, can be used if needed.

Babies and toddlers (6 months to 2 years): For this age group, a dilution ratio of 0.25-0.5%, or two to three drops of essential oil per ounce of carrier oil, works well.

Young Children (2–6 years): A 1% dilution, or 5–6 drops per ounce of carrier oil, is best for this age group.

For older kids (6–12 years old), a dilution ratio of 1–2% is good, which means 5–

10 drops of essential oil per ounce of carrier oil.

Women who are pregnant:

It is very important to be careful when using essential oils during pregnancy. It's usually safe to use 1% dilution, which is 5 to 6 drops of essential oil for every ounce of base oil. Some oils, like clary sage, rosemary, and some citrus oils, should not be used at all while you are pregnant.

4. Old people:

People over 65 may have skin that is thinner and more sensitive. An dilution ratio of 1% to 2% is usually safe. This means that 5 to 10 drops of essential oil should be mixed with 1 ounce of carrier oil. It's important to keep an eye out for any signs of soreness or sensitivity.

Places Not to Touch (like Eyes and Mucous Membranes)

It is important to avoid certain parts of the body when applying essential oils topically to avoid irritation and bad responses. You should stay away from the following places:

Eyes and Eyelids: The skin around your eyes is very sensitive, and essential oils can irritate, burn, and damage it badly. When you put oils near your eyes, be careful.

Mucous Membranes: You shouldn't put essential oils on mucous membranes like the inside of your nose, ears, mouth, or vaginal area. Because these tissues are so sensitive, the concentrated chemicals in essential oils can hurt them.

Broken or Damaged Skin: Unless your doctor tells you to, don't put essential oils on open wounds, cuts, or skin diseases like eczema or dermatitis. Essential oils can make discomfort worse and make it take longer to heal.

Skin Parts That Are More Sensitive: The neck, groin, and inner arms are some body parts that may be more sensitive to essential oils. If irritation happens, use lower dilution ratios or stay away from these places.

Sun-Exposed Areas: Some essential oils, like citrus oils like bergamot, lemon, and lime, are reactive, which means they can make the skin more likely to get burned in the sun. For 12 to 24 hours after putting these oils, don't put them on skin that will be in direct sunlight.

How often you use it

How often you use essential oils depends on what you want to do with them, how sensitive your skin is, and the type of oil you are using. Here are some general rules for how often you can use something safely:

Daily Use: Essential oils can be put on your face and body once a day for general health and beauty. Make sure the right amount of water is used, and keep an eye out for any soreness. For instance, you can use a diluted lavender oil mix every day to moisturize and calm your skin.

If you have an acute problem, like muscle pain, bug bites, or small skin irritations, you can use essential oils two to three times a day. But if you use it a lot, you should use lower dilution levels to keep your skin from becoming too sensitive.

Use Occasional: Essential oils can be used occasionally as needed to help with things like breathing problems or seasonal allergies. You can diffuse eucalyptus or peppermint oil several times a day to help clear up congestion, but you should only put it on your skin a few times a day at most.

Short-Term Use: If you want to use strong essential oils or oils that are more likely to make you sensitive, like oregano or cinnamon oil, only put them on your skin for a short time, like a few days to a week. When used for a long time, it can irritate and make skin more sensitive.

Monitoring and Making Changes: When using essential oils, it's important to keep an eye on the skin for any signs of swelling, irritation, itching, or pain. If any negative effects happen, stop using it right away and talk to a medical worker. Change the amount of dilution and how often you use it based on your own reactions and needs.

Rotating Oils: To lower the risk of sensitivity, you might want to use different essential oils every so often instead of the same oil all the time. This method gives the skin a chance to rest and lowers the chance of becoming sensitive to a certain oil.

Aromatherapy
Aromatherapy is a popular and effective way to use these powerful plant products. It involves using essential oils to improve your mental and physical health.
Essential oils can make a space relaxing, energizing, or therapeutic if they are used properly. Three important things to

keep in mind for safe and effective aromatherapy are how to use diffusers properly, making sure there is enough air flow and time, and learning how to mix essential oils.
Do not use in diffusers.

One Type of Diffusers Is:

Ultrasonic Diffusers: These diffusers use ultrasonic waves to turn the mixture of essential oil and water into a fine mist that is spread through the air. They are quiet, use little energy, and make the air more wet.

Nebulizing Diffusers: An air pump in these diffusers breaks up essential oils into tiny bits that are then released into the air. They don't need water and have a strong smell, so they can be used for healing purposes.

For evaporative diffusers, an air fan moves air through a pad or screen that has essential oils on it. The air flow makes the oil evaporate and spread all over the room. Even though they are easy to use, the oil might not be spread out as evenly as with other types.

With a heat diffuser, the essential oil is evaporated by heat. Even though they are quiet and can cover a big area, the heat can change the chemicals in the oils, which could make them less useful for healing.

2. How to Pick the Best Diffuser:

Choose a diffuser based on the size of the room and how strong of a flavor you want. Nebulizing diffusers are best for big rooms or therapeutic use, while ultrasonic diffusers work best in small to medium-sized rooms.

To keep mold and germs from growing, make sure the diffuser is easy to clean and maintain.

3. Guidelines for Correct Use:

To add water and essential oils, follow the directions on the package. Three to ten drops of essential oil are usually enough for most diffusers.

Do not overfill the diffuser, as this can cause it to stop working or work less well.

Regularly clean the diffuser by following the cleaning guidelines that came with it. Cleaning the diffuser on a regular basis keeps gunk from building up and makes sure it works well.

Keep the diffuser away from electronics and put it on a stable, flat surface. The mist can damage electronics.

Airflow and Length of Time
1. Making sure there is enough air flow:

It is very important to have enough air flow when spreading essential oils so that they don't overpower the senses.

In small or closed-off rooms, especially, open windows or doors to let air flow.

If you're using a diffuser in your bedroom, leave the door slightly open to let some air flow through and keep the essential oils from getting too concentrated.

2. How Long the Diffusion Lasts:

To get the most out of aromatherapy while minimizing the risk of overexposure, the length of diffusion should be carefully controlled.

A good rule of thumb is to breathe essential oils for 15 to 30 minutes at a time, two or three times a day. In this way, the body can absorb the good chemicals without becoming less sensitive or having bad affects.

If you want continuous diffusion, you might want to use a diffuser with intermittent settings, which switch between times of diffusion and rest (for example, 30 minutes on, 30 minutes off). This way can keep the therapeutic effects going longer without exposing too many people to them.

Watch how you and other people in the room feel during and after diffusion. If anyone is feeling pain, headaches, or dizziness, stop the diffusion and make sure there is enough air flow.

3. Things to think about for sensitive people:

People who have breathing problems, allergies, or sensitivities should be careful with aromatherapy. Use less concentrated essential oils and make sure there is plenty of air flow.

Essential oils may not be safe for pets, pregnant women, or young children. When they are around, only diffuse essential oils that are known to be safe for these groups in small amounts.

Putting together essential oils

1. How to Blend Well:

Blending essential oils means mixing different oils to make them work better together, which can improve their healing effects and give you a new scent experience.

When combining, think about what you want to happen. For instance, lavender, chamomile, and frankincense oils might be used in a blend to help you relax, while peppermint, eucalyptus, and lemon oils might be used in a mix to wake you up.

2. Types of Essential Oils:

Top Notes: These oils are light, clean, and healthy. They disappear quickly and are often the first smells that people notice when a blend is mixed. Citrus oils like lemon, lime, and bergamot, as well as peppermint and eucalyptus, are some examples.

Middle Notes: These oils give a mix balance and body. They don't evaporate very quickly and are usually found in the middle of a scent. Lavender, rosemary, and geranium are some examples.

Base Notes: These oils are rich, deep, and comforting. They slowly evaporate and give a mix depth that lasts.

Cedarwood, sandalwood, and patchouli are some examples.

3. Making a Blend That Is Balanced:

A well-balanced mix usually has the right amount of top, middle, and base notes for the effect and smell you want. A typical ratio is 3 parts top note, 2 parts middle note, and 1 part base note, but you can change it to suit your needs.

Start with a small amount and test the mix. If necessary, add more of each oil. Keep track of the amounts so that you can make the blend again later.

4. Thoughts on Safety:

When diffusing in a small area or for people who are sensitive, pay attention to how concentrated the essential oils are as a whole. To get the right amount of reduction, aim for 1-3% in the diffuser water.

To lower the risk of bad responses, don't mix oils that might have similar bad effects, like several oils that are known to make skin sensitive.

5. How to Store Blends:

Keep your essential oil mixes in dark glass bottles to keep them safe from light and keep them from going bad. Write the blend's name and the date it was made on the labels of the bottles.

Keep blends somewhere cool and dry to keep their strength and make them last longer.

Internal Use
When you use essential oils orally, you take them by mouth in small, controlled amounts to see if they help with your health. But this method is very debatable and comes with a lot of risks. Before thinking about this method, it's important to know about these risks, the debates about internal use, and how important it is to talk to a healthcare professional.
The risks and the debates

1. Possible Danger:

Essential oils are very concentrated plant products that contain strong chemicals. When these chemicals are taken by mouth, they can have strong effects on the body, both good and bad. Some essential oils have chemicals in them that are poisonous if eaten, even in small amounts. For instance, oils like eucalyptus and wintergreen contain chemicals that can hurt the liver and kidneys, cause seizures, or even kill you if you take them in the wrong way.

2. Problems with digestion:

When you eat or drink essential oils, they can irritate the lining of your digestive system. This irritation can show up as sickness, vomiting, diarrhea, or stomach pain. Peppermint and oregano oils are known to be strong and possibly irritating when taken by mouth, especially when they are taken in large amounts or without being reduced.

3. How Drugs Interact:

Essential oils can change how well medicines work or make side effects more likely when taken with other medicines. For example, oils like bergamot and grapefruit can mess up enzymes in the liver that break down some drugs. This can cause more of the drug to be in the blood, which increases the risk of overdose. People who are already taking medicines should be extra careful and talk to a doctor before consuming essential oils.

4. Effects on Allergies:

Some people may have allergic responses to certain essential oils if they eat or drink them. Some symptoms are mild, like itching or hives, and some are very bad, like anaphylactic. Before thinking about internal use, it's important to find possible allergens and know how sensitive you are to them.

5. Not enough rules:

In many countries, including the US, there are no rules about how essential oils can be used internally. As a result of this lack of control, there are no set rules for the safe amounts, purity, or quality of essential oils sold for internal use. Consumers have to rely on the image and honesty of the companies that make the goods, which can vary a lot.

6. Claims That Aren't True:

Some businesses and people may make claims about the benefits of taking essential oils that aren't true or aren't backed up by evidence. People may think that internal use is a cure-all because of these claims, but they don't fully understand the risks. It is important to think critically about these kinds of claims and look for information that is based on fact.

CHAPTER 5

Special Considerations

Use while breastfeeding and while pregnant

Extra care needs to be taken when using essential oils while pregnant or nursing because they could affect both the mother and the growing baby. Some oils are safe to use as long as they are used correctly, while others should never be used at all.

Which oils are safe and which ones you should stay away from

Safe Oils:

Lavandula angustifolia, or lavender, oil: Lavender oil is known to be calming and can help you sleep and feel less stressed. Most people think it's safe to use in moderation.

Frankincense oil (Boswellia carterii): This oil can help you relax and feel more grounded. It's safe to use while pregnant, and you can spread it out or dilute it before putting it on your skin.

Chamomile, also known as Matricaria chamomilla or Chamaemelum nobile, is a gentle plant that can help you relax and feel less anxious. On top of that, it can help with sickness.

Ginger, or Zingiber officinale,: Ginger oil can help with nausea and morning sickness. It can be spread around or put on the skin in a very weak form.

Lemon (Citrus limon): Lemon oil makes you feel good and clean. When spread or breathed in from a tissue, it can help lift your mood and make you feel less sick.

Oils you should stay away from:

Peppermint (Mentha piperita): Peppermint can help with sickness, but it can also make your uterus contract, so pregnant women should stay away from it.

Rosemary oil (Rosmarinus officinalis) can raise blood pressure and make the uterus contract, so it shouldn't be used while pregnant.

Clary Sage (Salvia sclarea): Clary sage is known to start labor, so pregnant women should stay away from it until later in the pregnancy.

Cinnamon: Cinnamon oil can be very sensitive to the skin and may have strong uterotonic effects, which means it could cause contractions.

Basil (Ocimum basilicum): If you are pregnant, you should stay away from basil oil because it can be too strong and irritate your skin.

The same level of care should be taken when feeding, because some essential oils can get into the milk and hurt the baby.

Oils that are safe for nursing:

Lavender can be used in small, weak amounts to help settle down.

Chamomile: It can help you relax, but don't use too much of it.

Tea Tree (Melaleuca alternifolia): Very small amounts of this oil can be used to kill germs.

Eucalyptus (Eucalyptus globulus): This plant can help with breathing, but it should only be used in small amounts and with care around babies.

Not to use these oils while nursing:

Peppermint: It can make you less likely to breastfeed and may give babies colic.

For some people, cinnamon is too strong and can irritate the skin.

Sage (Salvia officinalis) is known to make women less likely to have babies.

Wintergreen, or Gaultheria procumbens, has chemicals in it called salicylates that can be dangerous.

For use with babies and kids

Essential oils can be dangerous for kids and babies, so extra care needs to be taken to keep them safe. Always use the right amount of water to dilute essential oils, and only use ones that are thought to be safe for kids.

The Right Oils and Amounts

Safe Oils:

Lavender is gentle and relaxing, so it can be used with kids.

Chamomile is soothing, safe for kids, and can help them sleep and feel less anxious.

Tea Tree: Kills germs and can be used on skin problems with very small amounts.

Eucalyptus (Eucalyptus radiata): This is a milder type of eucalyptus that can help kids over 2 years old breathe better.

Frankincense is safe to use in small amounts and can help you feel calm and grounded.

How much to take:

For babies 0 to 6 months old, essential oils are usually not a good idea. If you need to, use just one drop mixed with two tablespoons of a neutral oil.

Babies and young children (6 months to 2 years): Mix 0.25 to 0.5% essential oil with 4 teaspoons of carrier oil. This is about 1 drop of essential oil per teaspoon of carrier oil.

For kids 2 to 6 years old, it's best to dilute the essential oil by 1%, which is about 1 drop of oil per teaspoon of carry oil.

For kids ages 6 to 12, a dilution of 1% to 2%, or 1-2 drops of essential oil per teaspoon of neutral oil, is fine.

Avoid these places:

Face and chest: Peppermint and eucalyptus oils work best here.

Hands: Kids can put their hands in their mouths or rub their eyes.

Skin That Is Broken or Damaged: Essential oils can irritate skin that is broken or damaged.

Use Near Pets

Essential oils can be harmful to pets, and some of them can even make them sick. When using essential oils around pets, it's important to be careful and know what could go wrong.

Possible dangers and safe ways to do things

Safe Oils:

Lavender is usually safe for dogs, and very small amounts can be used. It makes you feel better and can help with stress.

Chamomile is safe for dogs and can help them relax.

Frankincense is safe for dogs and can help with pain and stress.

Peppermint: Very little of this oil can be used on dogs, but cats should stay away from it.

Oils you should stay away from:

Tea Tree: Both cats and dogs can be seriously hurt by this plant.

Eucalyptus: Both cats and dogs can get sick from it.

Cats and dogs can both be irritated and hurt by cinnamon.

Dogs and cats should not be around citrus oils like lemon, orange, etc.

Wintergreen has chemicals in it that are like aspirin and can be harmful to cats.

How to Stay Safe:

Diluting: You should always dilute essential oils before putting them near pets. A safe range for dogs is between 0.5 and 1%.

Ventilation: When spreading essential oils, make sure the room has good air flow. This keeps the air clean and keeps you from getting too much sun.

Do Not Touch: Do not put essential oils on your pet's skin or fur directly. Instead, put them in a diffuser or make them very weak before putting them in places where your pet won't touch them.

When you give your pet a new essential oil, keep an eye out for any signs of distress or allergic responses. Keep an eye out for signs like drooling, feeling tired, throwing up, or having trouble breathing.

Talk to Your Vet: Before using essential oils on your pet, you should always talk to your vet, especially if your pet already has a health problem or is on medicine. When it comes to oils, a vet can tell you which ones are safe and how to use them correctly.

CHAPTER 6

Recognizing and Responding to Reactions

There are many good things about using essential oils, but it's also important to know about the bad things that can happen. If you notice these responses early on and act in the right way, you can help avoid bigger problems. There are common side effects, first aid steps, and advice on when to get medical help in this part.
Common Bad Side Effects

1. Itching of the skin:

Skin that is red, itchy, burning, or has a rash where the essential oil was applied.

When you put essential oils on your skin without diluting them first, when you use oils that are known to irritate the skin (like cinnamon or oregano), or when you have sensitive skin.

To keep yourself safe, always mix essential oils with a carrier oil before putting them on your skin. Before you use a new oil or blend, do a patch test. If you want to keep your skin healthy, don't use oils that are known to irritate it.

2. Effects on Allergies:

If you have hives, itching, swelling, or trouble breathing, it could mean that your allergic reaction is more serious.

Causes: Some people are sensitive to certain essential oils or parts of them.

In order to avoid getting sick, test any new essential oil on a small area of skin first. If you know you are allergic to something, talk to a doctor or nurse before using essential oils.

3. Damage from light:

Skin that is more sensitive to sunlight and gets sunburned or discolored when exposed to UV light.

When you put phototoxic oils on your skin, like citrus oils (bergamot, lemon, lime), and then leave it out in the sun, this happens.

To keep yourself safe, don't put phototoxic essential oils on skin that will be in direct sunlight. If you use these oils, make sure that the skin is covered or shielded from UV light for at least 12 to 24 hours.

4. Reactions in the lungs:

Signs: Coughing, sneezing, wheezing, or trouble breathing after taking in essential oils.

Reasons: Breathing in a lot of essential oils, especially in places with poor air flow, or using oils that can irritate the lungs, such as peppermint or eucalyptus.

Use essential oils in well-ventilated places and don't breathe in large amounts of them directly. If you have breathing problems like asthma, you should use smaller concentrations of oils when diffusing them.

5. Pain and fogginess in the head:

Headaches, feeling lightheaded, or dizzy after using essential oils are some of the symptoms.

Too much contact to strong smells or using oils that are too strong are two causes.

To avoid problems, only use a small amount of essential oils and make sure there is enough air flow. Start with small amounts and add more slowly if you need to.

How to Give First Aid

It is important to move right away to lessen the effects of a bad reaction if it happens. Here are some steps to take for first aid:

1. Itching of the skin:

Take Out the Oil: If the essential oil irritates your skin, wash the area right away with water and light soap to get rid of it.

Apply a carrier oil, such as coconut, almond, or olive oil, to the area that is hurt to help reduce the essential oil that is still on the skin.

Help the Skin Feel Better: To help the skin feel better, use a cool compress or aloe vera juice. Do not put any more essential oils on the area that is hurt.

2. Effects on Allergies:

Stop Using the Oil: Stop using the essential oil right away.

Wash the area with water and gentle soap to get rid of the oil.

Antacids: Antihistamines that you can buy over-the-counter can help ease the symptoms of mild allergic responses. Do what it says on the package of the medicine.

Get Medical Help: If your symptoms are serious, like having trouble breathing or your face or throat swelling up, you should get emergency medical help right away.

3. Damage from light:

Protect Your Skin: If you have used an essential oil that is phototoxic, cover your skin with clothes or put on sunscreen to keep it out of the sun.

Stay Out of the Sun: For at least 12 to 24 hours after using phototoxic oils, stay out of direct sunlight or take other protective steps.

Treat Sunburn: If phototoxicity caused the burn, use cool cloths, aloe vera gel, and over-the-counter sunburn medicines to heal the area.

4. Reactions in the lungs:

Get Some Fresh Air: If you're having breathing problems, get to a place with lots of fresh air and good air flow.

Stay hydrated: To help ease sore throats and lungs, drink water.

Seek Medical Help: If your respiratory problems are bad or don't get better, you should see a doctor right away.

5. Pain and fogginess in the head:

Stop Using the Oil: Stop using the essential oil and let some air flow through the space.

Rest: To help ease your symptoms, lie down in a room with good air flow and take deep breaths.

Stay hydrated: To stay hydrated, drink a lot of water.

Over-the-Counter Medicines: If you need to, use over-the-counter pain killers according to the directions on the bottle.

When you need to see a doctor

The majority of bad reactions to essential oils can be treated with first aid, but there are times when you need to see a doctor. To keep your health from getting worse, you should know when to get skilled help.

1. Strong reactions to allergies:

Signs: Having trouble breathing, face, lip, tongue, or throat swelling, a fast heart rate, or intense hives.

Take action: Get emergency medical help right away. If you are given one and can get one, use an epinephrine auto-injector (EpiPen).

2. Skin irritation that doesn't go away:

Symptoms: Redness, itching, or swelling that doesn't go away after first aid, or signs of an infection, like pus, more pain, or a fever.

Step 1: Seek help from a medical worker to get checked out and treated.

3. Signs of severe breathing problems:

Coughing, wheeze, trouble breathing, or chest tightness that doesn't get better with fresh air are all signs.

Take action: Seek medical help to check out and fix breathing problems.

4. Exposure to Eyes:

If essential oil gets in your eyes, you might feel burning, swelling, watering, or have trouble seeing.

Do something: Run cool water over your eyes for 15 to 20 minutes and then see a doctor.

5. Taking Essential Oils by Mouth:

If you take essential oils and then get sick, you might puke, feel sick, have stomach pain, become confused, or show other signs of toxicity.

What you should do is call a poison control center or go to the emergency room right away.

6. Reactions to light:

When you go outside after using phototoxic oils, you might get a severe sunburn, blisters, or skin discoloration.

Action: Seek medical help to get the right care and stop problems from getting worse.

CHAPTER 7

Responsible Sourcing and Purchasing

Responsible buying and sources are very important for using essential oils in a safe and useful way. Making sure the oils you buy are of good quality, reading labels and certifications, and picking items that are ethically and sustainably sourced are all important parts of having a good and safe experience.
How to Find Good Essential Oils

When choosing essential oils, quality is the most important thing. High-quality oils work better as medicine, are safer to use, and have more power. To help you find good essential oils, here are some tips:

1. Being pure:

100% Pure: Look for oils that say they are 100% pure essential oil and don't have any synthetic fillers, chemicals, or dilutions. Pure essential oils are the best because they keep the plant's natural qualities.

Botanical Name: The Latin name of the plant should be written on the sticker.

For instance, Lavandula angustifolia is the name of real lavender. This makes sure that you get the right oil and not a different one.

Country of Origin: The strength of the oil can be judged by where it comes from. Due to soil, temperature, and farming methods, plants grown in different areas have different make-ups. For example, the oil from Bulgarian lavender is very valuable.

2. Verification and Study:

GC/MS Testing: Gas Chromatography/Mass Spectrometry (GC/MS) testing is a popular way to find out what chemicals are in essential oils. Companies that offer GC/MS results show that they are honest and care about quality.

records for Each Batch: Reliable sellers usually give you GC/MS records that show the chemical makeup of the oil you're buying in each batch. This makes sure quality and regularity.

Third, smell and look:

Smell: Pure essential oils smell strong and natural. If an oil smells weak, too sweet, or fake, it might be fake or of low quality.

Color: Essential oils come in a range of colors, and some are thicker than others. Knowing the normal color and texture of certain oils can help you tell if they are pure. One good example of this is peppermint oil, which should be clear with a light yellow color.

Labels and Certifications: What They Mean

To make smart choices about the essential oils you buy, you need to be able to read and understand labels. Certifications can also give you peace of mind about quality and ethical sources.

1. Tags:

Plant Name and Common Name: The label should make it clear what the oil is called by both its common name and its plant name.

How the Oil Was Extracted: The label should say how the oil was extracted, such as by steam distillation or cold pressing. Different ways affect the quality of the oil and work better with some oils than others.

Parts Used: Saying what part of the plant was used (flowers, leaves, roots, etc.) can help you understand how the oil works.

Lot Number: A lot number, also called a batch number, makes it possible to track down an item and shows that the seller is well-organized.

Discontinuation Date: Essential oils don't really expire, but they can break down over time. An expiration date tells you how long the oil should stay at its strongest.

2. Proofs of identity:

Organic Certification: Look for organic approvals from well-known groups like Ecocert, the Soil Association, or USDA Organic. Synthetic pesticides, herbicides, and fertilizers are not used to make organic oils, so the result is purer.

This term, therapeutic grade, is used a lot in advertising, but it is not controlled by any group. Instead, look for oils that have been tried by independent labs and that are clear about where their ingredients come from and how they are made.

Fair Trade: If something is certified as Fair Trade, it means that the farms and other workers who help make it get paid fairly and are safe on the job. This approval also backs farming methods that are good for the environment.

Eco-Friendly and Responsible Sourcing

To protect the environment, help communities, and make sure that essential oils will be available for a long time, it is important to use ethical and healthy sourcing methods.

1. Effects on the environment:

Sustainable Harvesting: Plants that are used to make essential oils should be gathered in a way that doesn't harm the environment. Too much gathering can kill off plant species and hurt ecosystems. Look for suppliers who use harvesting ways that are good for the environment.

Wildcrafted Oils: These oils come from plants that were grown in the wild, where they belong. Make sure that wildcrafting is done in a way that doesn't hurt the environment or reduce the number of wild animals.

2. Helping out local communities:

Fair Wages: To source essential oils in an ethical way, you need to pay farmers and other workers who help grow and remove them fair wages. This is good for workers' quality of life and helps local businesses.

Community Projects: Some companies put money into community projects like building schools, hospitals, and clean water systems. By supporting these sellers, you help make the world a better place.

3. Partnering and getting certified:

Fair Trade Certification: As we already said, Fair Trade certification makes sure that businesses are doing the right thing when it comes to work and helping the community.

Partnerships with non-profits: Some businesses work with non-profits to make sure they source goods in an ethical and healthy way. A lot of the time, these partnerships include schooling, conservation projects, and building up communities.

4. Openness and being able to track:

Supplier Transparency: Reliable sellers should tell you about their supply chain, such as where and how the plants are grown, harvested, and processed.

Traceability: Being able to find out where the oil came from makes sure that it is pure and safe. Often, batch numbers and clear communication from the seller can prove this.

5. Stay away from endangered species:

Protection Level: Know the protection level of plants that are used to make essential oils. Don't use oils that come from species that are threatened or rare. Protected species are governed by groups such as CITES (Convention on International Trade in Endangered Species of Wild Fauna and Flora).

Alternatives: If the original plant is in danger, choose other essential oils that have similar effects. As an example, you could use amyris oil instead of sandalwood, which is in danger of going extinct, because it is found in a way that doesn't harm the environment.

THE END